The Quick and Easy Pegan Diet Cookbook for Beginners

Start your Weight Loss Journey and Look Beautiful with Super Tasty and Vibrant Pegan Diet Recipes

Emy Fit

© Copyright 2020 - All rights reserved.

The content contained within this book may not be reproduced, duplicated or transmitted without direct written permission from the author or the publisher.

Under no circumstances will any blame or legal responsibility be held against the publisher, or author, for any damages, reparation, or monetary loss due to the information contained within this book. Either directly or indirectly.

Legal Notice:

This book is copyright protected. This book is only for personal use. You cannot amend, distribute, sell, use, quote or paraphrase any part, or the content within this book, without the consent of the author or publisher.

Disclaimer Notice:

Please note the information contained within this document is for educational and entertainment purposes only. All effort has been executed to present accurate, up to date, and reliable, complete information. No warranties of any kind are declared or implied. Readers acknowledge that the author is not engaging in the rendering of legal, financial, medical or professional advice. The content within this book has been derived from various sources. Please consult a licensed professional before attempting any techniques outlined in this book.

By reading this document, the reader agrees that under no circumstances is the author responsible for any losses, direct or indirect, which are incurred as a result of the use of information contained within this document, including, but not limited to, — errors, omissions, or inaccuracies.

Table of Contents

Fresh Black Bean Dip 9
Easy Vegan Quest Dip 11
Vegan Seven-Layer Dip 12
Chocolate Chip Peanut Butter Dip 15
Air-Fried Tofu 16
Green Chili Hummus with Salsa 17
Crostini with Pecan Basil Pesto 19
Black-Eyed Pea Dip 21
Caramelized Onion Hummus 22
Spicy Roasted Chickpeas 24
Southwestern Hummus 25
Vegan Bacon Ricotta Crostini 27
Vegan Beer Brats in a Blanket 29
Baked Jalapeño Poppers 31
Vegan Spinach Cheese Pinwheels 33
Cocktail Lentil Meatballs 35
Carrot Hummus 37
Vegan Cheesy Popcorn 39
Easy Vegan Rangoon Dip 41
Tapas Made of Swan and Hummus 43
Keto Coconut Flake Balls 45
Tofu Nuggets with Cilantro Dip 47
Keto Chocolate Greek Yoghurt Cookies 48
Bacon-Wrapped Sausage Skewers 50
Bacon-Wrapped Mozzarella Sticks 51
Broiled Bacon Wraps with Dates 52
Caramelized Bacon Knots 53
Chocolate Dipped Candied Bacon 54
Tropical Coconut Balls 56

Jicama Fries	58
Ham 'n' Cheese Puffs	59
Beet Balls	61
Cheesy Crackers	63
Tomato Soup	65
Meatballs Platter	67
Quick Zucchini Bowl	69
Healthy Basil Platter	71
Spiced Vegetable Couscous	73
Pasta e Fagioli with Orange and Fennel	75
Spaghetti al Limone	78
Spiced Baked Rice with Fennel	80
Yogurt Dip	82
Tomato Bruschetta	85
Artichoke Flatbread	86
Red Pepper Tapenade	88
Coriander Falafel	89
Red Pepper Hummus	91
White Bean Dip	93
Hummus with Ground Lamb	94
Bulgur Lamb Meatballs	95
Eggplant Dip	97
Veggie Fritters	98
Cucumber Bites	99
Stuffed Avocado	100
Wrapped Plums	101
Cucumber Sandwich Bites	102
Cucumber Rolls	103
Olives and Cheese Stuffed Tomatoes	104
Vinegar Beet Bites	105

Lentils Stuffed Potato Skins.. 106

Fresh Black Bean Dip

Preparation time: 5 minutes

Cooking time: 30 minutes

Servings: 5

Ingredients:

- 1 small yellow onion, peeled and chopped
- 2 jalapeño peppers
- 1 clove garlic, peeled and chopped
- 1/4 cup red bell pepper
- 2 (15-ounce) cans black beans, drained
- 3 tablespoons water
- 1 teaspoon ground cumin
- 2 teaspoons cocoa powder
- 3 tablespoons fresh lime juice
- 2 tablespoons fresh chopped cilantro
- 4 cherry tomatoes, sliced

Directions:

1. Add onion, jalapeño, garlic, bell pepper, black beans, and water to a food processor bowl. Pulse three times, pushing down contents that go up sides of bowl. Add cumin and cocoa powder and pulse again until smooth.
2. Pour into a medium microwave-safe container and cook 60 seconds. Stir and repeat. Remove from microwave and let cool 1 minute.
3. Stir in lime juice and cilantro. Cover and refrigerate up to 5 days or freeze up to 2 months. To serve, cook in microwave in 30-second intervals until heated through, then garnish with sliced cherry tomatoes.

Nutrition:

Calories: 88

Fat: 0.3 g
Protein: 5.5 g
Sodium: 191 mg
Fiber: 6.5 g
Carbohydrates: 18.9 g
Sugar: 1.4 g

Easy Vegan Quest Dip

Preparation time: 5 minutes

Cooking time: 15minutes

Servings: 6

Ingredients:

- 1 (8-ounce) package vegan cream cheese
- 1 (10-ounce) can mild green chili enchilada sauce
- 3 tablespoons nutritional yeast flakes
- 1 teaspoon garlic powder
- 1/2 teaspoon salt
- 1/4 teaspoon black pepper

Directions:

1. Scoop vegan cream cheese into a small microwave-safe bowl and microwave about 20 seconds. Remove, stir, and repeat until sauce is smooth and stirs easily.
2. Pour green chili enchilada sauce over cream cheese. Stir to combine. Stir in nutritional yeast flakes, garlic powder, salt, and pepper. Let cool about 5 minutes before covering and refrigerating up to 7 days.
3. To serve, remove from refrigerator and cook in microwave in 30-second intervals until heated through.

Nutrition: Calories: 78 Fat: 0.3 g Protein: 2.5 g Sodium: 191 mg Fiber: 5.5 g Carbohydrates: 19.9 g Sugar: 1.4 g

Vegan Seven-Layer Dip

Preparation time: 5 minutes

Cooking time: 15minutes

Servings: 10

Ingredients:

- 1 (12-ounce) package vegan meat crumbles
- 1 tablespoon olive oil
- 3 tablespoons taco seasoning
- 1 can black beans
- 1.1/2 cups mild chunky salsa, divided
- 2 cups vegan Cheddar shreds
- 1 cup vegan sour cream
- 1 cup guacamole
- 1 (2.25-ounce) can black olives, chopped
- 1/2 cup chopped tomatoes
- 1/2 cup chopped green onion

Directions:

1. In a large skillet, brown vegan meat crumbles in olive oil over medium heat about 5 minutes. Add taco seasoning. Set aside to cool to room temperature, about 5 minutes.
2. Place beans in a blender or food processor with 1/2 cup salsa. Blend about 20 seconds until beans are consistency of refried beans.
3. Spread beans into bottom of a large serving tray that is about 11/2" deep. Sprinkle shredded cheese on top of beans. Sprinkle vegan meat crumbles on top of cheese. Carefully spread sour cream on top of vegan crumbles, and then spread guacamole on top of sour cream. Pour remaining salsa over guacamole and spread evenly. Sprinkle with olives. Garnish with tomatoes and green onions. Cover and refrigerate up to 3 days.

Nutrition:
Calories: 58
Fat: 3.3 g
Protein: 2.5 g
Carbohydrates: 19.9 g
Sugar: 1.4 g

Chocolate Chip Peanut Butter Dip

Preparation time: 5 minutes

Cooking time: 10minutes

Servings: 10

Ingredients:

- 1 (15-ounce) can chickpeas, rinsed and drained
- 3/4 cup creamy peanut butter
- 1/2 cup agave nectar
- 1 teaspoon vanilla extract
- 3 tablespoons filtered water
- 1 cup dairy-free chocolate chips

Directions:

1. Pour all ingredients except chocolate chips into bowl of a food processor.
2. Pulse 3 seconds. Use a spatula to push down ingredients from sides of bowl. Pulse an additional 40 seconds.
3. Transfer to a small lidded container and stir in chocolate chips. Store in refrigerator up to 5 days.

Nutrition: Calories: 79 Fat: 7.3 g Protein: 4.5 g Sodium: 191 mg Fiber: 8.5 g Carbohydrates: 20.9 g Sugar: 1.4 g

Air-Fried Tofu

Preparation time: 5 minutes

Cooking time: 15minutes

Servings: 4

Ingredients:

- 1 (15-ounce) package extra-firm tofu, pressed and cut into 1/2" cubes
- 2 teaspoons olive oil
- 1/4 teaspoon salt

Directions:

1. Preheat air fryer to 375°F and set timer for 18 minutes. Allow air fryer to heat up 30 seconds. Remove fryer basket and spray with vegetable cooking spray. Add tofu cubes and olive oil. Toss to coat, then place basket back in air fryer.
2. Every 5 minutes, remove basket and stir tofu by shaking basket carefully. Cook until timer goes off and tofu is crispy. Remove from basket and sprinkle with salt.
3. Let cool 10 minutes, then transfer tofu to a large sealed container and refrigerate up to 5 days.
4. To serve, reheat tofu in the air fryer heated at 350°F for 5 minutes.

Nutrition: Calories: 49 Fat: 8.3 g Protein: 4.5 g Sodium: 191 mg Fiber: 8.5 g Carbohydrates: 20.9 g Sugar: 1.4 g

Green Chili Hummus with Salsa

Preparation time: 5 minutes

Cooking time: 15minutes

Servings: 12

Ingredients:

- 1 (15-ounce) can chickpeas, rinsed and drained
- 2 tablespoons tahini
- 2 tablespoons nutritional yeast flakes
- 2 teaspoons garlic powder
- 1 (4-ounce) can green chilies
- 1/2 cup fresh spinach
- 1 (8-ounce) jar mild chunky salsa

Directions:

1. Combine chickpeas, tahini, nutritional yeast flakes, garlic powder, green chilies, and spinach in a food processor. Pulse 3 seconds until coarse and crumbly.
2. Set a colander and pour salsa into colander to strain liquid.
3. Add liquid 1 tablespoon at a time to food processor and pulse until a spreadable consistency is reached.
4. Spoon hummus into a small serving dish and top with strained salsa.
5. Cover and keep refrigerated until ready to serve (up to 4 days). Alternatively, it can be frozen up to 1 month.
6. *Serve and enjoy.*

Nutrition:

Calories: 69

Fat: 8.3 g

Protein: 4.5 g

Sodium: 121 mg

Fiber: 6.5 g
Carbohydrates: 20.9 g
Sugar: 1.4 g

Crostini with Pecan Basil Pesto

Preparation time: 5 minutes

Cooking time: 15minutes

Servings: 8

Ingredients:

- 1/3 cup pecans
- 1 cup fresh spinach
- 1/3 cup olive oil
- 2 teaspoons vegan Parmesan
- 1 teaspoon garlic powder
- 5 fresh basil leaves
- 1 baguette, sliced into 24 (1/2"-thick) slices

Directions:

1. Set oven and place pecans on an ungreased baking sheet and toast in oven about 5 minutes. Remove and cool about 2 minutes.
2. Place cooled pecans, spinach, olive oil, vegan Parmesan, garlic powder, and basil leaves in a food processor. Pulse 3 seconds to combine.
3. Set bread slices in one layer on a large ungreased baking sheet. Place in oven and toast about 5 minutes. Remove from oven and cool about 5 minutes, then transfer to a medium sealed container and refrigerate up to 3 days.
4. To serve, wrap toast with foil and heat in toaster oven at 350°F for 5 minutes, until heated through. Top with Pecan Basil Pesto.

Nutrition:

Calories: 65

Fat: 2.3 g

Protein: 9.5 g

Sodium: 121 mg

Fiber: 6.5 g
Carbohydrates: 14.9 g
Sugar: 1.4 g

Black-Eyed Pea Dip

Preparation time: 5 minutes

Cooking time: 35minutes

Servings: 6

Ingredients:

- 1 (15-ounce) can black eye peas, drained
- 3 tablespoons finely chopped peeled yellow onion
- 1/4 cup vegan sour cream
- 1/2 (8-ounce) jar mild chunky salsa
- 1 cup vegan Cheddar shred.

Directions:

1. Place black eye peas in an ungreased 8" × 8" casserole dish and use a fork to mash up most of beans.
2. Add in onions, sour cream, salsa, and 1/2 vegan Cheddar shreds. Stir to combine. Top mixture with remaining vegan Cheddar shreds.
3. Bake 25 minutes until top cheese layer melts. Remove from oven and allow to cool 15 minutes.
4. Transfer dip to a large sealable container and refrigerate up to 5 days. To serve, cook in microwave in 30-second intervals until heated through.

Nutrition:

Calories: 55

Fat: 2.3 g

Protein: 9.5 g

Sodium: 111 mg

Fiber: 6.5 g

Carbohydrates: 18.9 g

Sugar: 1.4 g

Caramelized Onion Hummus

Preparation time: 5 minutes

Cooking time: 35minutes

Servings: 10

Ingredients:

- 1 small yellow onion
- 3 tablespoons olive oil, divided
- 1 teaspoon agave nectar
- 1 (15-ounce) can chickpeas, rinsed and drained
- 1/4 cup pine nuts
- 3 tablespoons lime juice
- 1/2 teaspoon dried basil
- 1 tablespoon nutritional yeast flakes
- 1 clove garlic, peeled

Directions:

1. Set a skillet on a low heat and add onions. Drizzle with 1 tablespoon olive oil. Cook until tender, about 5 minutes. Then add agave nectar and continue cooking about 10 minutes, until caramelized. Remove from heat and set aside.
2. Add chickpeas into a food processor with pine nuts and pulse 5 seconds. Add remaining tablespoons olive oil, lime juice, basil, nutritional yeast flakes, garlic, and 1/2 caramelized onions. Pulse 3 seconds until smooth. Top with remaining caramelized onions. Transfer to a medium lidded container and refrigerate up to 5 days.

Nutrition:

Calories: 79

Fat: 8.3 g

Protein: 17.5 g

Sodium: 231 mg
Fiber: 6.5 g
Carbohydrates: 18.9 g
Sugar: 1.4 g

Spicy Roasted Chickpeas

Preparation time: 5 minutes

Cooking time: 35minutes

Servings: 4

Ingredients:

- 1 can chickpeas
- 11/2 teaspoons olive oil
- 1 tablespoon Southwest Chipotle seasoning
- 1/2 teaspoon salt
- 1/8 teaspoon ground black pepper

Directions:

1. Preheat oven to 400°F.
2. Add chickpeas and olive oil to a medium bowl and stir until each chickpea is coated with oil. Place chickpeas on prepared pan.
3. Bake 25 minutes until chickpeas are crispy on outside.
4. Remove from oven and sprinkle seasoning over top. Stir until thoroughly coated. Sprinkle with salt and pepper, then transfer to a small sealed container and refrigerate up to 5 days.

Nutrition:

Calories: 56

Fat: 8.3 g

Protein: 15.5 g

Sodium: 121 mg

Fiber: 6.5 g

Carbohydrates: 18.9 g

Sugar: 1.4 g

Southwestern Hummus

Preparation time: 5 minutes

Cooking time: minutes

Servings: 10

Ingredients:

- 1 (15-ounce) can chickpeas, rinsed and drained
- 1/4 cup tahini
- 1/4 cup lime juice
- 1 cup mild chunky salsa
- 1 tablespoon Southwest Chipotle seasoning

Directions:

1. Pour all ingredients in bowl of food processor and pulse 3 seconds. Use a spatula to scrape down any ingredients on side of bowl. Pulse again until consistency is smooth.
2. Transfer to a small sealed container and refrigerate up to 5 days.

Nutrition:

Calories: 56

Fat: 8.3 g

Protein: 15.5 g

Sodium: 121 mg

Fiber: 6.5 g

Carbohydrates: 18.9 g

Sugar: 1.4 g

Vegan Bacon Ricotta Crostini

Preparation time: 5 minutes

Cooking time: 10 minutes

Servings: 10

Ingredients:

- 1 baguette, cut into 24 slices
- 1 tablespoon olive oil
- 1 clove garlic, peeled and chopped
- 8 slices vegan bacon
- 1 cup cashews
- 1/2 cup unsweetened almond milk
- 1 tablespoon nutritional yeast flakes
- 1 teaspoon dried basil
- 1 tablespoon mild miso paste
- 1/4 cup maple syrup

Directions:

1. Preheat oven to 375°F. Set a baking sheet.
2. Set slices on prepared baking sheet and bake 10 minutes until toasted. Transfer to a large sealable bag and refrigerate up to 5 days.
3. Place a medium skillet over medium heat. Add olive oil and garlic. Set aside.
4. In same skillet, cook vegan bacon 3 minutes per side. Take off from skillet and set aside to cool about 5 minutes, and then break into pieces.
5. Add soaked cashews, almond milk, nutritional yeast flakes, basil, and miso paste to bowl of food processor. Pulse 3 seconds. Repeat process until mixture is smooth and leaves no large pieces of cashews.

6. Transfer to a medium sealable container and refrigerate up to 5 days. To serve, top each piece of toasted crostini with one dollop cashew ricotta, followed by divided-out vegan bacon pieces and maple syrup. Toast in toaster oven at 300°F for 5 minutes until crispy.

Nutrition:

Calories: 56

Fat: 8.3 g

Protein: 15.5 g

Fiber: 6.5 g

Carbohydrates: 18.9 g

Sugar: 1.4 g

Vegan Beer Brats in a Blanket

Preparation time: 5 minutes

Cooking time: 20minutes

Servings: 10

Ingredients:

- 1/4 cup yellow mustard
- 1 tablespoon agave nectar
- 1 (12-ounce) bottle pale lager beer
- 4 vegan brats
- 8 dairy-free crescent rolls
- 1 cup dill and garlic sauerkraut
- 1 cup vegan mozzarella cheese
- 4 slices vegan bacon, halved

Directions:

1. Preheat oven to 350F.
2. Combine mustard and agave nectar in a small lidded bowl. Cover and refrigerate up to 7 days.
3. Pour beer into a medium saucepan and bring to a boil over medium heat. Add brats and cook. Once processed, cut each brat in half. Set aside.
4. Arrange dough pieces on prepared baking sheet, adding sauerkraut and vegan cheese evenly over each.
5. Wrap each brat piece in 1/2 slice vegan bacon. Place on piece of dough. Wrap dough tightly around each brat and pinch to seal dough. Bake 15 minutes.
6. Let rolls cool 10 minutes, then transfer to a large lidded container and refrigerate up to 5 days. To serve, remove from refrigerator and heat in microwave in 30-second intervals until heated through. Pour mustard sauce over each roll.

Nutrition:

Calories: 56
Fat: 8.3 g
Protein: 15 g
Sodium: 12 mg
Fiber: 6 g
Carbohydrates: 18.g
Sugar: 1.4 g

Baked Jalapeño Poppers

Preparation time: 5 minutes

Cooking time: 20minutes

Servings: 10

Ingredients:

- 1/2 (8-ounce) container dairy-free cream cheese, softened
- 1/2 (14.2-ounce) container Diana Jalapeño Garlic Havarti Style Wedge, shredded
- 3/4 cup + 1 tablespoon plain soy milk, divided
- 1/8 teaspoon garlic powder
- 1/2 teaspoon salt
- 10 jalapeños, halved and seeded
- 2 tablespoons ground flaxseed
- 1/2 cup all-purpose flour
- 1/2 cup bread crumbs

Directions:

1. Preheat oven to 350°F.
2. Place vegan cream cheese, shredded vegan cheese, 1 tablespoon soy milk, garlic powder, and salt in a medium bowl and stir until well combined. Stuff each halved jalapeño with an even amount cream cheese mixture.
3. In a separate medium bowl combine flaxseed and remaining soy milk. Set aside.
4. Pour flour into a small dish and bread crumbs into another. Set aside.
5. Roll a stuffed jalapeño in flour, and then dip in flaxseed mixture, followed by a final dip in bread crumbs. Place breaded popper on prepared pan and repeat dipping process with remaining stuffed jalapeños.

6. *Take out from oven and let cool. Transfer to a large sealed container and refrigerate up to 5 days. To serve, heat in a toaster oven at 350°F for about 5 minutes.*

Nutrition:

Calories: 12

Fat: 873 g

Protein: 12 g

Sodium: 12 mg

Fiber: 6 g

Carbohydrates: 18.g

Sugar: 1.4 g

Vegan Spinach Cheese Pinwheels

Preparation time: 15 minutes

Cooking time: 0minutes

Servings: 10

Ingredients:

- 1/2 cup shredded vegan jack cheese
- 1/4 cup vegan Parmesan cheese
- 2 tablespoons chopped green onion
- 1/4 teaspoon garlic powder
- 1/2 teaspoon salt
- 1/4 cup all-purpose flour
- 1 Pepperidge Farm Puff Pastry Sheet
- 1 tablespoon vegan butter, melted
- 1 tablespoon plain soy milk
- 1 package frozen chopped spinach

Directions:

1. In a medium bowl stir together vegan cheeses, green onions, garlic powder, and salt.
2. Prepare a work area by sprinkling with flour. Lay out pastry sheet on floured surface. Stir together melted vegan butter and soy milk in a small bowl and brush over top of pastry sheet, reserving remaining mixture.
3. Spread cheese mixture over buttered pastry sheet, and then spread drained spinach over cheese mixture.
4. Begin with side closest to you and roll pastry sheet, wrapping ingredients in as you roll. Wrap pastry roll in aluminum foil and freeze about 30 minutes.
5. Preheat oven to 400°F. Grease a baking sheet with vegetable cooking spray.

6. Use a serrated knife to cut pastry roll into 1/2" slices. Place slices on prepared pan and brush with reserved butter mixture.
7. Bake 20 minutes until pinwheels are a golden color.
8. Remove from oven and let cool about 5 minutes before transferring to a large sealed container. Refrigerate up to 5 days. To serve, cook in a toaster oven at 350°F until heated through, about 5 minutes.

Nutrition:

Calories: 10

Fat: 873 g

Protein: 121g

Sodium: 16 mg

Fiber: 6 g

Carbohydrates: 18.g

Sugar: 1.4 g

Cocktail Lentil Meatballs

Preparation time: 15 minutes

Cooking time: 25minutes

Servings: 9

Ingredients:

- 1 cup chopped peeled yellow onion
- 1 cup dried brown lentils
- 3 cups water
- 1 cup extra-firm tofu, pressed
- 2 tablespoons ground flaxseed, divided
- 11/4 cups rolled oats, divided
- 1 tablespoon cashews
- 2 teaspoons Better than Bouillon Seasoned Vegetable Base
- 1 tablespoon nutritional yeast flakes
- 1 teaspoon rubbed sage
- 1/4 teaspoon ground turmeric
- 1 teaspoon paprika
- 3/4 cup grape jelly
- 11/2 cups ketchup
- 1 teaspoon sriracha

Directions:

1. Add onions, lentils, and water to a small saucepan. Bring to a boil over high heat, then reduce heat to low, cover, and cook 25 minutes. Strain excess liquid and set aside.
2. In a food processor add tofu, 1 tablespoon flaxseed, and 1/2 cup rolled oats, cashews, better than Bouillon, nutritional yeast flakes, sage, turmeric, and paprika. Pulse until combined.

3. Add 2 cups strained lentil mixture to tofu mixture. Pulse to combine. Add remaining lentil mixture and use a spatula to stir. Add remaining flaxseed and oats and stir to combine. Set aside about 5 minutes to allow mixture to thicken.
4. Preheat oven to 375°F. Line two baking sheets with parchment paper.
5. Use a cookie dough scoop to measure consistent portions from mixture. Form into balls.
6. Place lentil meatballs on prepared pans, allowing some space between them.
7. Bake 25 minutes, turning over once, halfway through bake. When lentil meatballs are done, remove from oven and let cool about 10 minutes.
8. To prepare sauce, combine grape jelly, ketchup, and sriracha in a large microwave-safe bowl. Heat in microwave 30 seconds then stir. Repeat heating until jelly has melted and a sauce form. Add meatballs to sauce, stirring gently to coat.
9. Transfer meatballs to a large lidded container and refrigerate up to 5 days, or freeze up to 2 months.

Nutrition: Calories: 10 Fat: 30 g Protein: 121g Sodium: 16 mg Fiber: 6 g Carbohydrates: 18.g Sugar: 1.4 g

Carrot Hummus

Preparation time: 15 minutes

Cooking time: 0minutes

Servings: 9

Ingredients:

- 1 (15-ounce) can chickpeas, rinsed and drained
- 1 cup roughly chopped peeled carrots
- 1 tablespoon balsamic vinegar
- 2 teaspoons garlic powder
- 1/2 teaspoon ground cumin
- 1/2 teaspoon ground turmeric
- 1 teaspoon dried basil
- 1 tablespoon tamari
- 2 tablespoons all-natural peanut butter
- 4 tablespoons water
- 2 tablespoons olive oil

Directions:

1. Place all ingredients except water and olive oil in a food processor and pulse until combined. Remove lid and stir ingredients, adding water 1 tablespoon at a time until desired consistency is reached.
2. Transfer to a medium lidded container and refrigerate up to 7 days. To serve, drizzle olive oil on top of hummus.

Nutrition:

Calories: 9

Fat: 20 g

Protein: 11g

Sodium: 16 mg

Fiber: 6 g

Carbohydrates: 18.g
Sugar: 1.4 g

Vegan Cheesy Popcorn

Preparation time: 5 minutes

Cooking time: 5minutes

Servings: 2

Ingredients:

- 1/3 cup popcorn kernels
- 2 teaspoons nutritional yeast flakes
- 1 teaspoon paprika
- 1/2 teaspoon ground turmeric
- 1/8 teaspoon salt

Directions:

1. Place popcorn kernels in a microwave popcorn popper. Place lid on container and microwave about 3minutes.
2. Place nutritional yeast flakes, paprika, and turmeric in a small bowl. Stir to combine.
3. Use oven mitts to remove popcorn popper from microwave, then carefully remove lid.
4. Pour popcorn into a large sealable container, removing unpeopled kernels. Spray popcorn generously with vegetable cooking spray. Sprinkle nutritional yeast mixture and salt over top and use your hands or a spoon to distribute seasonings evenly throughout popcorn.

Nutrition:

Calories: 9

Fat: 19 g

Protein: 11g

Sodium: 15 mg

Fiber: 6 g

Carbohydrates: 18.g

Sugar: 1.4 g

Easy Vegan Rangoon Dip

Preparation time: 5 minutes

Cooking time: 15minutes

Servings: 10

Ingredients:
- 1 cup Frank's Red-hot Sweet Chili Sauce
- 1 (15-ounce) container extra-firm tofu, pressed and cut into 1/2" cubes
- 1 (8-ounce) container vegan cream cheese, divided
- 1 green onion, chopped
- About 10 tortilla chips, crushed

Directions:
1. Preheat oven to 350°F.
2. Pour sauce in a medium skillet over medium heat. Add tofu and allow simmering in sauce 3 minutes. Be sure to stir tofu well while cooking. Use a spatula to break up tofu more.
3. Add 2 tablespoons cream cheese to tofu mixture and stir to incorporate. Remove from heat and set aside.
4. Spread remaining cream cheese in bottom of a 1.5-quart casserole dish. Top with green onions. Pour tofu and sauce over cream cheese and top with crushed tortilla chip pieces.
5. Bake 25 minutes, then remove from oven and let cool about 10 minutes.
6. Cover and refrigerate up to 7 days. To serve, let sit until room temperature or heat in microwave in 30-second intervals until heated through.

Nutrition:

Calories: 9

Fat: 17 g

Protein: 17g
Sodium: 10 mg
Fiber: 6 g
Carbohydrates: 18.g
Sugar: 1.4 g

Tapas Made of Swan and Hummus

Preparation time: 5 minutes

Cooking time: 15minutes

Servings: 6

Ingredients:

- 2/3 cup quinoa
- 1 cup vegetable cups
- 1/2 tsp. paprika
- 1/2 teaspoon chili powder with fries
- 1-teaspoon garlic powder
- 1 tsp. onion
- 1-cup cornstarch and one ear
- 1 cooked chickpea with a cup
- Divide 1 cup cherry tomatoes into wedges
- 2 tablespoons of lime juice
- 1/2 kosher or a teaspoon of salt to taste
- 1 tablespoon Spinach leaves
- 6 milk cakes (giant burrito)

Directions:

1. Always cook quinoa before cooking. Place the winch in a bowl with enough water to cover about an inch. Rub the quinoa seriously into your hands. The water becomes cloudy with sapiens; the layer of protective seeds disappears bitterly. Repeat three times, then rinse under running water. I use eye compression.
2. Combine quinoa, broth, paprika, pepper, garlic, and onion in a small saucepan over medium heat. Heat for 20 minutes, envelope, reduce heat and cool. You know the grain is ready in the package.

3. Pour quinoa into a large bowl and mix with corn, beans, tomatoes, and lemon juice. Salt to taste.
4. Spread the hummus on all types of mulch, gently cover the spinach leaves, and add about 1/3 of the casino quinoa mix in the center. Turn the other side of the turkey onto a crannog and wrap it tightly. Close the toothbrush.

Nutrition:

Calories: 9

Fat: 19 g

Protein: 17g

Sodium: 101mg

Fiber: 6 g

Carbohydrates: 187g

Sugar: 1.4 g

Keto Coconut Flake Balls

Preparation Time: 15 Minutes

Cooking Time: 0 Minutes

Servings: 2

Ingredients:

- 1 Vanilla shortbread collagen protein bar
- 1 tablespoon lemon
- ¼ teaspoon ground ginger
- ½ cup unsweetened coconut flakes,
- ¼ teaspoon ground turmeric

Directions:

1. Process protein bar, ginger, turmeric, and ¾ of the total flakes into a food processor.
2. Remove and add a spoon of water and roll till dough forms.
3. Roll into balls, and sprinkle the rest of the flakes on it. Serve.

Nutrition:

Calories: 204 kcal

Total Fat: 11g

Total Carbs: 4.2g

Protein: 1.5g

Tofu Nuggets with Cilantro Dip

Preparation Time: 10 Minutes

Cooking Time: 15 Minutes

Servings: 4

Ingredients:

- 1 lime, ½ juiced and ½ cut into wedges
- 1½ cups olive oil
- 28 oz tofu, pressed and cubed
- 1 egg, lightly beaten
- 1 cup golden flaxseed meal
- 1 ripe avocado, chopped
- ½ tablespoon chopped cilantro
- Salt and black pepper to taste
- ½ tablespoon olive oil

Directions:

1. Heat olive oil in a deep skillet. Coat tofu cubes in the egg and then in the flaxseed meal. Fry until golden brown. Transfer to a plate.
2. Place avocado, cilantro, salt, pepper, and lime juice in a blender; puree until smooth. Spoon into a bowl, add tofu nuggets, and lime wedges to serve.

Nutrition:

Calories: 665

Net Carbs: 6.2g

Fat: 54g

Protein: 32g

Keto Chocolate Greek Yoghurt Cookies

Preparation Time: 15 Minutes

Cooking Time: 30 Minutes

Servings: 3

Ingredients:

- 3 eggs
- 1/8 teaspoon tartar
- 5 tablespoons softened Greek yogurt

Directions:

1. Beat the egg whites, the tartar, and mix.
2. In the yolk, put in the Greek yogurt, and mix.
3. Combine both egg whites and yolk batter into a bowl.
4. Bake for 25-30 minutes, serve.

Nutrition:

Calories: 287 kcal

Total Fat: 19g

Total Carbs: 6.5g

Protein: 6.8g

Bacon-Wrapped Sausage Skewers

Preparation Time: 10 Minutes

Cooking Time: 8 Minutes

Servings: 4

Ingredients:
- 5 Italian chicken sausages
- 10 slices bacon

Directions:

1. Preheat the deep fryer to 370°F/190°C
2. Cut the sausage into four pieces.
3. Slice the bacon in half.
4. Wrap the bacon over the sausage.
5. Skewer the sausage.
6. Fry for 4-5 minutes until browned.
7. Remove from the fryer and serve hot.

Nutrition:

Calories: 331 kcal

Protein: 11.84 g

Fat: 30.92 g

Carbohydrates: 1.06g

Bacon-Wrapped Mozzarella Sticks

Preparation Time: 5 Minutes

Cooking Time: 5 Minutes

Servings: 2

Ingredients:

- 2 slices thick bacon
- 2 Frigo® Cheese Heads String Cheese sticks
- Coconut oil – for frying
- For Dipping: Low-sugar pizza sauce

Directions:

1. Warm the oil to 350º Fahrenheit in a deep fryer.
2. Slice the cheese stick in half. Wrap it with the bacon and close it using the toothpick.
3. Cook the sticks in the hot fryer for two to three minutes
4. Drain on a towel and cool. Serve with sauce.

Nutrition:

Calorie Count: 103

Protein: 7 g

Fat: 9 g

Carbohydrates: 1 g

Broiled Bacon Wraps with Dates

Preparation Time: 10 Minutes

Cooking Time: 20 Minutes

Servings: 6

Ingredients:

- 1 lb. sliced bacon
- 8 oz. pitted dates

Directions:

1. Heat the oven to reach 425° Fahrenheit.
2. Use a ½ slice of bacon and wrap each of the dates. Close with a toothpick.
3. Put the wraps on a baking tray and bake them for 15-20 minutes. Serve hot.

Nutrition:

Calorie: 203

Protein: 19 g

Fats: 10 g

Carbohydrates: 5 g

Caramelized Bacon Knots

Preparation Time: 10 Minutes

Cooking Time: 15 Minutes

Servings: 4

Ingredients:

- 8 sliced bacon
- 1 tablespoon black pepper
- 1 tablespoon Low-carb sweetener - your preference

Directions:

1. Mix the pepper blend and sweetener in a small bowl. Set aside.
2. Slice each bacon slice in half. Tie each half into a knot.
3. Press the bacon knots into the pepper mixture, turning them over to coat as much as possible. Place the dipped knots onto a wire rack placed on a baking tin.
4. Place the bacon knots under a hot broiler and cook until they're to your liking (5-7 min. per side).
5. Cool on a layer of paper towels to remove excess grease as needed.
6. Serve as soon as they're ready.

Nutrition:

Calorie Count: 187

Protein: 5 g

Fat: 17 g

Carbohydrates: 1 g

Chocolate Dipped Candied Bacon

Preparation Time: 20 Minutes

Cooking Time: 1 Hour 15 Minutes

Servings: 6

Ingredients:

- ½ teaspoon Cinnamon
- 2 tablespoon brown sugar alternative – ex. Surkin Gold
- 16 thin-cut slices of bacon
- ½ oz. cacao butter or coconut oil
- 3 oz. 85% dark chocolate
- 1 teaspoon Sugar-free maple extract

Directions:

1. Whisk the Surkin Gold and cinnamon together.
2. Arrange the bacon strips on a parchment paper-lined tray and sprinkle using half of the mixture. Do the other side with the rest of the seasoning mixture.
3. Set the oven to reach 275° Fahrenheit. Bake until caramelized and crispy (approximately 1 hour and 15 minutes).
4. Heat a skillet to melt the cocoa butter and chocolate. Pour the maple syrup into the mixture and stir well. Set aside until it's room temperature.
5. Arrange the bacon on a platter to cool thoroughly before dipping it into the chocolate.
6. Dip half of each strip of the bacon into the chocolate.
7. Arrange on a tray for the chocolate to solidify. Either place it in the refrigerator or on the countertop.

Nutrition:

Calorie Count: 54

Protein: 3 g

Fat: 4.1 g

Carbohydrates: 1.1 g

Tropical Coconut Balls

Preparation Time: 15 Minutes

Cooking Time: 20 Minutes

Servings: 2

Ingredients:

- 1 cup shredded coconut (unsweetened)
- 6 tablespoons coconut milk (full-fat)
- 2 tablespoons melted coconut oil
- 1/4 cup almond flour
- 2 tablespoons lemon juice
- 2 tablespoons ground chia seeds
- Zest of 1 lemon
- 10 drops stevia (alcohol-free)
- 1/8 teaspoons sea salt

Directions:

1. Preheat the oven to 250 degrees Fahrenheit
2. Place the shredded coconut in a large bowl and pour the coconut milk into it.
3. Add the almond flour, ground chia, sea salt, coconut oil, and lemon zest, and lemon juice to the bowl.
4. Mix everything until well combined.
5. Take 1 tablespoon of the mixture and form a ball out of it. Repeat with the remaining mixture.
6. Line a baking tray using parchment paper and place the small balls on it.
7. If you find the mixture too dry while making the balls, add one tablespoon (extra) of coconut oil to the mixture
8. Bake the coconut balls for 30 minutes and remove them from the oven.
9. Let it cool completely at room temperature.
10. Transfer the balls into another container carefully and refrigerate it for 30 minutes.
11. Serve chilled and enjoy!

Nutrition:

Calories 134 Kcal
Fat: 13.1 g
Protein: 2.2 g
Net carb: 1.1 g

Jicama Fries

Preparation Time: 5 Minutes

Cooking Time: 10 Minutes
Servings: 2

Ingredients:

- 1 Jicama (sliced into thin strips)
- 1/2 teaspoon onion powder
- 2 tablespoons avocado oil
- Cayenne pepper (pinch)
- 1 teaspoon paprika
- Sea salt, to taste

Directions:

1. Dry roast the jicama strips in a non-stick frying pan (or you can also grease the pan with a bit of avocado oil)
2. Place the roasted jicama fries into a large bowl and add the onion powder, cayenne pepper, paprika, and sea salt.
3. Drizzle over the avocado oil and toss the contents until the flavors are incorporated well.
4. Serve immediately and enjoy!

Nutrition:

Calories 92 Kcal

Fat: 7 g

Protein: 1 g

Net carb: 2 g

Ham 'n' Cheese Puffs

Preparation Time: 15 Minutes
Cooking Time: 30 Minutes
Servings: 8
Ingredients:

- 6 large eggs
- 10 oz. sliced deli ham, diced
- 1 ½ cup shredded cheddar cheese
- ¾ cup mayonnaise
- 1/3 cup coconut flour
- 1/3 cup coconut oil
- 1/3 teaspoon baking powder
- 1/3 teaspoon baking soda
- Nonstick cooking spray

Directions:

1. Set the oven to 350°F. Lightly coat rimmed baking sheet using nonstick cooking spray and set aside.
2. In a bowl, put together the eggs, coconut oil, and mayonnaise. Mix and set aside.
3. In a separate bowl, combine the baking soda, baking powder, and coconut flour. Add the dry ingredients to the wet ingredients and mix well until smooth.
4. Fold the ham and cheddar cheese into the mixture and set aside.
5. Cut the dough into 18 small pieces then arrange on the prepared baking sheet.
6. Bake for 30 minutes, or until the puffs are golden brown and set.
7. Arrange the puffs on a cooling rack and allow to cool slightly.
8. Store it in a sealed container for up to 5 days. If desired, reheat in the microwave before serving.

Nutrition:

Calories: 249

Fat: 20g
Carbs: 3g
Protein: 15g

Beet Balls

Preparation Time: 10 Minutes

Cooking Time: 0 Minutes

Servings: 6

Ingredients:

- ½ cup oats

- 1 medium beet, cooked

- ½ cup almond flour

- 1/3 cup shredded coconut and more for coating

- ¾ cup Medjool dates, pitted

- 1 tablespoon cocoa powder

- ½ cup peanuts

- ¼ cup chocolate chips, unsweetened

Directions:

1. Place cooked beets in a blender and then pulse until chopped into very small pieces.
2. Add remaining ingredients and then pulse until the dough comes together.
3. Shape the dough into eighteen balls, coat them in some more coconut and then serve.

Nutrition:

Calories: 114.2 Cal;

Fat: 2.4 g;

Protein: 5 g;

Carbs: 19.6 g;

Fiber: 4.9 g

Cheesy Crackers

Preparation Time: 10 Minutes

Cooking Time: 20 Minutes

Servings: 3

Ingredients:

- 1 ¾ cup almond meal
- 3 tablespoons nutritional yeast
- ½ teaspoon of sea salt
- 2 tablespoons lemon juice
- 1 tablespoon melted coconut oil
- 1 tablespoon ground flaxseed
- 2 ½ tablespoons water

Directions:

1. Switch on the oven, then set it to 350 degrees F and let it preheat.
2. Meanwhile, take a medium bowl, place flaxseed in it, stir in water, and then let the mixture rest for 5 minutes until thickened.
3. Place almond meal in a medium bowl, add salt and yeast and then stir until mixed.
4. Add lemon juice and oil into the flaxseed mixture and then whisk until mixed.

5. Pour the flaxseed mixture into the almond meal mixture and then stir until dough comes together.

6. Place a piece of a wax paper on a clean working space, place the dough on it, cover with another piece of wax paper, and then roll dough into a 1/8-inch-thick crust.

7. Cut the dough into a square shape, sprinkle salt over the top and then bake for 15 to 20 minutes until done.

8. Serve straight away.

Nutrition:

Calories: 30 Cal;

Fat: 1 g;

Protein: 1 g;

Carbs: 5 g;

Fiber: 0 g

Tomato Soup

Preparation Time: 10 Minutes

Cooking Time: 10 Minutes

Servings: 2

Ingredients:

- 56 ounces stewed tomatoes
- ¼ teaspoon salt
- ¼ teaspoon ground black pepper
- 1 medium red bell pepper, cored, diced
- ¼ teaspoon dried thyme
- 6 leaves of basil, chopped
- ¼ teaspoon dried oregano
- 1 teaspoon olive oil

Directions:

1. Take a medium pot, place it over medium heat, add oil, and when hot, add bell pepper and then cook for 4 minutes.
2. Add remaining ingredients into the pot, stir until mixed, switch heat to medium-high heat, and bring the mixture to simmer.
3. Remove pot from the heat and then puree the soup until smooth.

4. Taste to adjust seasoning, ladle soup into bowls and then serve.

Nutrition:

Calories: 170 Cal;

Fat: 1.1 g;

Protein: 3.5 g;

Carbs: 36 g;

Fiber: 2.6 g

Meatballs Platter

Preparation Time: 10 Minutes

Cooking Time: 15 Minutes

Servings: 4

Ingredients:
- 1-pound beef meat, ground
- ¼ cup panko breadcrumbs
- A pinch of salt and black pepper
- 3 tablespoons red onion, grated
- ¼ cup parsley, chopped
- 2 garlic cloves, minced
- 2 tablespoons lemon juice
- Zest of 1 lemon, grated
- 1 egg
- ½ teaspoon cumin, ground
- ½ teaspoon coriander, ground
- ¼ teaspoon cinnamon powder
- 2 ounces feta cheese, crumbled
- Cooking spray

Directions:

1. In a bowl, blend the beef with the breadcrumbs, salt, pepper and the rest of the ingredients except the cooking spray, stir well and shape medium balls out of this mix.
2. Arrange the meatballs on a baking sheet lined with parchment paper, grease them with cooking spray and bake at 450 degrees F for 15 minutes.
3. Position the meatballs on a platter and serve as a snack.

Nutrition:

Calories: 300,

Fat: 15.4,

Fiber: 6.4,

Carbs: 22.4,

Protein: 35

Quick Zucchini Bowl

Preparation Time: 10 Minutes

Cooking Time: 10 Minutes

Servings: 4

Ingredients:

- ½ pound of pasta
- 2 tablespoons of olive oil
- 6 crushed garlic cloves
- 1 teaspoon of red chili
- 2 finely sliced spring onions
- 3 teaspoons of chopped rosemary
- 1 large zucchini cut up in half, lengthways and sliced
- 5 large portabella mushrooms
- 1 can of tomatoes
- 4 tablespoons of Parmesan cheese
- Fresh ground black pepper

Directions:
1. Cook the pasta.
2. Take a large-sized frying pan and place over medium heat.

3. Add oil and allow the oil to heat up.
4. Add garlic, onion and chili and sauté for a few minutes until golden.
5. Add zucchini, rosemary and mushroom and sauté for a few minutes.
6. Increase the heat to medium-high and add tinned tomatoes to the sauce until thick.
7. Drain your boiled pasta and transfer to a serving platter.
8. Pour the tomato mix on top and mix using tongs.
9. Garnish with Parmesan cheese and freshly ground black pepper.
10. Enjoy!

Nutrition:

Calories: 361

Fat: 12g

Carbohydrates: 47g

Protein: 14g

Healthy Basil Platter

Preparation Time: 25 Minutes

Cooking Time: 15 Minutes

Servings: 4

Ingredients:

- 2 pieces of red pepper seeded and cut up into chunks
- 2 pieces of red onion cut up into wedges
- 2 mild red chilies, diced and seeded
- 3 coarsely chopped garlic cloves
- 1 teaspoon of golden caster sugar
- 2 tablespoons of olive oil (plus additional for serving)
- 2 pounds of small ripe tomatoes quartered up
- 12 ounces of dried pasta
- Just a handful of basil leaves
- 2 tablespoons of grated Parmesan

Directions:

1. Pre-heat the oven to 392 degrees Fahrenheit.
2. Take a large-sized roasting tin and scatter pepper, red onion, garlic and chilies.

3. Sprinkle sugar on top.
4. Drizzle olive oil then season with pepper and salt.
5. Roast the veggies in your oven for 15 minutes.
6. Take a large-sized pan and cook the pasta in boiling, salted water until Al Dente.
7. Drain them.
8. Remove the veggies from the oven and tip in the pasta into the veggies.
9. Toss well and tear basil leaves on top.
10. Sprinkle Parmesan and enjoy!

Nutrition:

Calories: 452

Fat: 8g

Carbohydrates: 88g

Protein: 14g

Spiced Vegetable Couscous

Preparation Time: 10 minutes

Cooking Time: 20 minutes

Servings: 2

Ingredients

- Cauliflower – 1 head, cut into 1 –inch florets
- Extra-virgin olive oil – 6 tbsp. plus extra for serving
- Salt and pepper
- Couscous – 1 ½ cups
- Zucchini – 1, cut into ½ inch pieces
- Red bell pepper – 1, stemmed, seeded, and cut into ½ inch pieces
- Garlic – 4 cloves, minced
- Ras el hanout – 2 tsp.
- Grated lemon zest -1 tsp. plus lemon wedges for serving
- Chicken broth – 1 ¾ cups
- Minced fresh marjoram – 1 tbsp.

Directions

1. In a skillet, heat 2 tbsp. oil over medium heat.

2. Add cauliflowers, ¾ tsp. salt, and ½ tsp. pepper. Mix.
3. Cover and cook for 5 minutes, or until the florets start to brown and the edges are just translucent.
4. Remove the lid and cook, stirring for 10 minutes, or until the florets turn golden brown. Transfer to a bowl and clean the skillet.
5. Heat 2 tbsp. oil in the skillet.
6. Add the couscous. Cook and stir for 3 to 5 minutes, or until grains are just beginning to brown. Transfer to a bowl and clean the skillet.
7. Heat the remaining 3 tbsp. oil in the skillet and add bell pepper, zucchini, and ½ tsp. salt. Cook for 6 to 8 minutes, or until tender.
8. Stir in lemon zest, ras el hanout, and garlic. Cook until fragrant (about 30 seconds).
9. Stir in the broth and bring to a simmer.
10. Stir in the couscous. Cover, remove from the heat, and set aside until tender (about 7 minutes).
11. Add marjoram and cauliflower; then gently fluff with a fork to combine.
12. Drizzle with extra oil and season with salt and pepper.
13. Serve with lemon wedges.

Nutrition

Calories: 787

Fat: 18.3g

Carb: 129.6g

Protein: 24.5g

Pasta e Fagioli with Orange and Fennel

Preparation Time: 10 minutes

Cooking Time: 30 minutes

Servings: 5

Ingredients

- Extra-virgin olive oil – 1 tbsp. plus extra for serving
- Pancetta – 2 ounces, chopped fine
- Onion – 1, chopped fine
- Fennel – 1 bulb, stalks discarded, bulb halved, cored, and chopped fine
- Celery – 1 rib, minced
- Garlic – 2 cloves, minced
- Anchovy fillets – 3, rinsed and minced
- Minced fresh oregano – 1 tbsp.
- Grated orange zest – 2 tsp.
- Fennel seeds – ½ tsp.
- Red pepper flakes – ¼ tsp.
- Diced tomatoes – 1 (28-ounce) can
- Parmesan cheese – 1 rind, plus more for serving
- Cannellini beans – 1 (7-ounce) cans, rinsed

-
- Chicken broth – 2 ½ cups
- Water – 2 ½ cups
- Salt and pepper
- Orzo – 1 cup
- Minced fresh parsley – ¼ cup

Directions

1. Heat oil in a Dutch oven over medium heat. Add pancetta.
2. Stir-fry for 3 to 5 minutes or until beginning to brown.
3. Stir in celery, fennel, and onion and stir-fry until softened (about 5 to 7 minutes).
4. Stir in pepper flakes, fennel seeds, orange zest, oregano, anchovies, and garlic. Cook for 1 minute.
5. Stir in tomatoes and their juice. Stir in Parmesan rind and beans.
6. Bring to a simmer and cook for 10 minutes.
7. Stir in water, broth, and 1 tsp. salt.
8. Increase heat to high and bring to a boil.
9. Stir in pasta and cook for 10 minutes, or until al dente.
10. Remove from heat and discard parmesan rind.
11. Stir in parsley and season with salt and pepper to taste.
12. Drizzle with olive oil and sprinkle with grated Parmesan.
13. Serve.

Nutrition

Calories: 502

Fat: 8.8g

Carb: 72.2g

Protein: 34.9g

Spaghetti al Limone

Preparation Time: 10 minutes

Cooking Time: 15 minutes

Servings: 2

Ingredients

- Extra-virgin olive oil – ½ cup
- Grated lemon zest – 2 tsp.
- Lemon juice – 1/3 cup
- Garlic – 1 clove, minced to pate
- Salt and pepper
- Parmesan cheese – 2 ounces, grated
- Spaghetti – 1 pound
- Shredded fresh basil – 6 tbsp.

Directions

1. In a bowl, whisk garlic, oil, lemon zest, juice, ½ tsp. salt and ¼ tsp. pepper. Stir in the Parmesan and mix until creamy.
2. Meanwhile, cook the pasta according to package directions. Drain and reserve ½ cup cooking water.
3. Add the oil mixture and basil to the pasta and toss to combine.

4. Season with salt and pepper to taste and add the cooking water as needed.

5. Serve.

Nutrition:

Calories: 398

Fat: 20.7g

Carb: 42.5g

Protein: 11.9g

Spiced Baked Rice with Fennel

Preparation Time: 10 minutes

Cooking Time: 45 minutes

Servings: 2

Ingredients

- Sweet potatoes – 1 ½ pounds, peeled and cut into 1-inch pieces
- Extra-virgin olive oil – ¼ cup
- Salt and pepper
- Fennel – 1 bulb, chopped fine
- Small onion – 1, chopped fine
- Long-grain white rice – 1 ½ cups, rinsed
- Garlic – 4 cloves, minced
- Ras el hanout – 2 tsp.
- Chicken broth – 2 ¾ cups
- Large pitted brine-cured green olives – ¾ cup, halved
- Minced fresh cilantro – 2 tbsp.
- Lime wedges

Directions

1. Adjust the oven rack to the middle position and heat the oven to 400F. Toss the potatoes with ½ tsp. salt and 2 tbsp. oil.

2. Arrange the potatoes in a single layer in a rimmed baking sheet and roast for 25 to 30 minutes, or until tender. Stir the potatoes halfway through roasting.
3. Remove the potatoes from the oven and lower the oven temperature to 350F.
4. In a Dutch oven, heat the remaining 2 tbsp. oil over medium heat.
5. Add onion and fennel; next, cook for 5 to 7 minutes, or until softened. Stir in ras el hanout, garlic, and rice. Stir-fry for 3 minutes.
6. Stir in the olives and broth and let sit for 10 minutes. Add the potatoes to the rice and fluff gently with a fork to combine.
7. Season with salt and pepper to taste.
8. Sprinkle with cilantro and serve with lime wedges.

Nutrition

Calories: 207

Fat: 8.9g

Carb: 29.4g

Protein: 3.9g

Yogurt Dip

Preparation Time: 10 Minutes
Cooking Time: 0 Minutes
Servings: 6
Ingredients:

- 2 cups Greek yogurt
- 2 tablespoons pistachios, toasted and chopped
- A pinch of salt and white pepper
- 2 tablespoons mint, chopped
- 1 tablespoon kalamata olives, pitted and chopped
- ¼ cup za'atar spice
- ¼ cup pomegranate seeds
- 1/3 cup olive oil

Directions:

1. In a bowl, blend the yogurt with the pistachios and the rest of the ingredients, whisk well.
2. Divide into small cups and serve with pita chips on the side.

Nutrition:

Calories: 294,

Fat: 18,

Fiber: 1,
Carbs: 21,

Protein: 10

Tomato Bruschetta

Preparation Time: 10 Minutes
Cooking Time: 10 Minutes
Servings: 6
Ingredients:

- 1 baguette, sliced
- 1/3 cup basil, chopped
- 6 tomatoes, cubed
- 2 garlic cloves, minced
- A pinch of salt and black pepper
- 1 teaspoon olive oil
- 1 tablespoon balsamic vinegar
- ½ teaspoon garlic powder
- Cooking spray

Directions:

1. Arrange the baguette slices in the baking sheet lined with parchment paper, grease them with cooking spray and bake at 400 degrees F for 10 minutes.
2. In a bowl, mix the tomatoes with the basil and the remaining ingredients, toss well and leave aside for 10 minutes.
3. Divide the tomato mix on each baguette slice, arrange them all on a platter and serve.

Nutrition:

Calories: 162,

Fat: 4,

Fiber: 7,

Carbs: 29,

Protein: 4

Artichoke Flatbread

Preparation Time: 10 Minutes
Cooking Time: 15 Minutes
Servings: 4
Ingredients:

- 5 tablespoons olive oil
- 2 garlic cloves, minced
- 2 tablespoons parsley, chopped
- 2 round whole wheat flatbreads
- 4 tablespoons parmesan, grated
- ½ cup mozzarella cheese, grated
- 14 ounces canned artichokes, drained and quartered
- 1 cup baby spinach, chopped
- ½ cup cherry tomatoes, halved
- ½ teaspoon basil, dried
- Salt and black pepper to the taste

Directions:

1. In a bowl, mix the parsley with the garlic and 4 tablespoons oil, whisk well and spread this over the flatbreads.
2. Sprinkle the mozzarella and half of the parmesan.
3. In a bowl, mix the artichokes with the spinach, tomatoes, basil, salt, pepper and the rest of the oil, toss and divide over the flatbreads as well.
4. Sprinkle the remaining of the parmesan on top, arrange the flatbreads on a baking sheet lined with parchment paper and bake at 425 degrees F for 15 minutes.
5. Serve a snack.

Nutrition:

Calories: 223,

Fat: 11.2,

Fiber: 5.34,

Carbs: 15.5,

Protein: 7.4

Red Pepper Tapenade

Preparation Time: 10 Minutes
Cooking Time: 0 Minutes
Servings: 4
Ingredients:

- 7 ounces roasted red peppers, chopped
- ½ cup parmesan, grated
- 1/3 cup parsley, chopped
- 14 ounces canned artichokes, drained and chopped
- 3 tablespoons olive oil
- ¼ cup capers, drained
- 1 and ½ tablespoons lemon juice
- 2 garlic cloves, minced

Directions:

1. In your blender, combine the red peppers with the parmesan and the rest of the ingredients and pulse well.
2. Divide into cups and serve as a snack.

Nutrition:

Calories: 200,

Fat: 5.6,

Fiber: 4.5,

Carbs: 12.4,

Protein: 4.6

Coriander Falafel

Preparation Time: 10 Minutes
Cooking Time: 10 Minutes
Servings: 8
Ingredients:

- 1 cup canned garbanzo beans, drained and rinsed
 1 bunch parsley leaves
- 1 yellow onion, chopped
- 5 garlic cloves, minced
- 1 teaspoon coriander, ground
- A pinch of salt and black pepper
- ¼ teaspoon cayenne pepper
- ¼ teaspoon baking soda
- ¼ teaspoon cumin powder
- 1 teaspoon lemon juice
- 3 tablespoons tapioca flour
- Olive oil for frying

Directions:

1. In your food processor, combine the beans with the parsley, onion and the rest the ingredients except the oil and the flour and pulse well.
2. Transfer the mix to a bowl, add the flour, stir well, shape 16 balls out of this mix and flatten them a bit.
3. Heat up a pan with some oil over medium-high heat, add the falafels, cook them for 5 minutes on each side, transfer to paper towels, drain excess grease, arrange them on a platter and serve as an appetizer.

Nutrition:

Calories: 112,

Fat: 6.2,

Fiber: 2,

Carbs: 12.3,

Protein: 3.1

Red Pepper Hummus

Preparation Time: 10 Minutes
Cooking Time: 0 Minutes
Servings: 6
Ingredients:

- 6 ounces roasted red peppers, peeled and chopped
- 16 ounces canned chickpeas, drained and rinsed
- ¼ cup Greek yogurt
- 3 tablespoons tahini paste
- Juice of 1 lemon
- 3 garlic cloves, minced
- 1 tablespoon olive oil
- A pinch of salt and black pepper
- 1 tablespoon parsley, chopped

Directions:

1. In your food processor, combine the red peppers with the rest of the ingredients except the oil and the parsley and pulse well.
2. Add the oil, pulse again, divide into cups, sprinkle the parsley on top and serve as a party spread.

Nutrition:

Calories: 255,

Fat: 11.4,

Fiber: 4.5,

Carbs: 17.4,

Protein: 6.5

White Bean Dip

Preparation Time: 10 Minutes
Cooking Time: 0 Minutes
Servings: 4
Ingredients:

- 15 ounces canned white beans
- 6 ounces canned artichoke hearts, drained and quartered
- 4 garlic cloves, minced
- 1 tablespoon basil, chopped
- 2 tablespoons olive oil
- Juice of ½ lemon
- Zest of ½ lemon, grated
- Salt and black pepper to the taste

Directions:

1. In your food processor, combine the beans with the artichokes and the rest of the ingredients except the oil and pulse well.
2. Add the oil gradually, pulse the mix again, divide into cups and serve as a party dip.

Nutrition:

Calories: 274,

Fat: 11.7,

Fiber: 6.5,

Carbs: 18.5,

Protein: 16.5

Hummus with Ground Lamb

Preparation Time: 10 Minutes

Cooking Time: 15 Minutes

Servings: 8

Ingredients:

- 10 ounces hummus
- 12 ounces lamb meat, ground
- ½ cup pomegranate seeds
- ¼ cup parsley, chopped
- 1 tablespoon olive oil
- Pita chips for serving

Directions:

1. Heat up a pan with the oil over medium-high heat, add the meat, and brown for 15 minutes stirring often.
2. Spread the hummus on a platter, spread the ground lamb all over, also spread the pomegranate seeds and the parsley and serve with pita chips as a snack.

Nutrition:

Calories: 133,

Fat: 9.7,

Fiber: 1.7,

Carbs: 6.4,

Protein: 5.4

Bulgur Lamb Meatballs

Preparation Time: 10 Minutes
Cooking Time: 15 Minutes
Servings: 6
Ingredients:

- 1 and ½ cups Greek yogurt
- ½ teaspoon cumin, ground
- 1 cup cucumber, shredded
- ½ teaspoon garlic, minced
- A pinch of salt and black pepper
- 1 cup bulgur
- 2 cups water
- 1-pound lamb, ground
- ¼ cup parsley, chopped
- ¼ cup shallots, chopped
- ½ teaspoon allspice, ground
- ½ teaspoon cinnamon powder
- 1 tablespoon olive oil

Directions:

1. In a bowl, blend the bulgur with the water, cover the bowl, leave aside for 10 minutes, drain and transfer to a bowl.
2. Add the meat, the yogurt and the rest of the ingredients except the oil, stir well and shape medium meatballs out of this mix.
3. Heat up a pan with the oil over medium-high heat, add the meatballs, cook them for 7 minutes on each side, arrange them all on a platter and serve as a snack.

Nutrition:

Calories: 300,

Fat: 9.6,

Fiber: 4.6,

Carbs: 22.6,

Protein: 6.6

Eggplant Dip

Preparation Time: 10 Minutes

Cooking Time: 40 Minutes

Servings: 4

Ingredients:

- 1 eggplant, poked with a fork
- 2 tablespoons tahini paste
- 2 tablespoons lemon juice
- 2 garlic cloves, minced
- 1 tablespoon olive oil
- Salt and black pepper to the taste
- 1 tablespoon parsley, chopped

Directions:

1. Put the eggplant in a roasting pan, bake at 400 degrees F for 40 minutes, cool down, peel and transfer to your food processor.
2. Add the rest of the fixings excluding the parsley, pulse well, divide into small bowls and serve as a snack with the parsley sprinkled on top.

Nutrition:

Calories: 121,

Fat: 4.3,

Fiber: 1,

Carbs: 1.4,

Protein: 4.3

Veggie Fritters

Preparation Time: 10 Minutes

Cooking Time: 10 Minutes

Servings: 8

Ingredients:

- 2 garlic cloves, minced
- 2 yellow onions, chopped
- 4 scallions, chopped
- 2 carrots, grated
- 2 teaspoons cumin, ground
- ½ teaspoon turmeric powder
- Salt and black pepper to the taste
- ¼ teaspoon coriander, ground
- 2 tablespoons parsley, chopped
- ¼ teaspoon lemon juice
- ½ cup almond flour
- 2 beets, peeled and grated
- 2 eggs, whisked
- ¼ cup tapioca flour
- 3 tablespoons olive oil

Directions:

1. In a bowl, combine the garlic with the onions, scallions and the rest of the ingredients except the oil, stir well and shape medium fritters out of this mix.
2. Heat up a pan with the oil on medium-high heat, add the fritters, cook for 5 minutes on each side, arrange on a platter and serve.

Nutrition:

Calories: 209,

Fat: 11.2,

Fiber: 3,

Carbs: 4.4,

Protein: 4.8

Cucumber Bites

Preparation Time: 10 Minutes

Cooking Time: 0 Minutes

Servings: 12
Ingredients:

- 1 English cucumber, sliced into 32 rounds
- 10 ounces hummus
- 16 cherry tomatoes, halved
- 1 tablespoon parsley, chopped
- 1-ounce feta cheese, crumbled

Directions:

1. Spread the hummus on each cucumber round, divide the tomato halves on each, sprinkle the cheese and parsley on to and serve as a snack.

Nutrition:

Calories: 162,

Fat: 3.4,

Fiber: 2,

Carbs: 6.4,

Protein: 2.4

Stuffed Avocado

Preparation Time: 10 Minutes

Cooking Time: 0 Minutes

Servings: 2

Ingredients:

- 1 avocado, halved and pitted
- 10 ounces canned tuna, drained
- 2 tablespoons sun-dried tomatoes, chopped
- 1 and ½ tablespoon basil pesto
- 2 tablespoons black olives, pitted and chopped
- Salt and black pepper to the taste
- 2 teaspoons pine nuts, toasted and chopped
- 1 tablespoon basil, chopped

Directions:

1. In a bowl, blend the tuna with the sun-dried tomatoes and the rest of the ingredients except the avocado and stir.
2. Stuff the avocado halves with the tuna mix and serve as a snack.

Nutrition:

Calories: 233,

Fat: 9,

Fiber: 3.5,

Carbs: 11.4,

Protein: 5.6

Wrapped Plums

Preparation Time: 5 Minutes

Cooking Time: 0 Minutes

Servings: 8

Ingredients:

- 2 ounces prosciutto, cut into 16 pieces
- 4 plums, quartered
- 1 tablespoon chives, chopped
- A pinch of red pepper flakes, crushed

Directions:

1. Wrap each plum quarter in a prosciutto slice, arrange them all on a platter, sprinkle the chives and pepper flakes all over and serve.

Nutrition:

Calories: 30,

Fat: 1,

Fiber: 0,

Carbs: 4,

Protein: 2

Cucumber Sandwich Bites

Preparation Time: 5 Minutes

Cooking Time: 0 Minutes

Servings: 12

Ingredients:

- 1 cucumber, sliced
- 8 slices whole wheat bread
- 2 tablespoons cream cheese, soft
- 1 tablespoon chives, chopped
- ¼ cup avocado, peeled, pitted and mashed
- 1 teaspoon mustard
- Salt and black pepper to the taste

Directions:

1. Spread the mashed avocado on each bread slice, also spread the rest of the ingredients except the cucumber slices.
2. Divide the cucumber slices on the bread slices, cut each slice in thirds, arrange on a platter and serve as a snack.

Nutrition:

Calories: 187,

Fat: 12.4,

Fiber: 2.1,

Carbs: 4.5,

Protein: 8.2

Cucumber Rolls

Preparation Time: 5 Minutes

Cooking Time: 0 Minutes

Servings: 6

Ingredients:
- 1 big cucumber, sliced lengthwise
- 1 tablespoon parsley, chopped
- 8 ounces canned tuna, drained and mashed
- Salt and black pepper to the taste
- 1 teaspoon lime juice

Directions:
1. Arrange cucumber slices on a working surface, divide the rest of the ingredients, and roll.
2. Arrange all the rolls on a platter and serve as a snack.

Nutrition:

Calories: 200,

Fat: 6,

Fiber: 3.4,

Carbs: 7.6,

Protein: 3.5

Olives and Cheese Stuffed Tomatoes

Preparation Time: 10 Minutes

Cooking Time: 0 Minutes

Servings: 24

Ingredients:

- 24 cherry tomatoes, top cut off and insides scooped out
- 2 tablespoons olive oil
- ¼ teaspoon red pepper flakes
- ½ cup feta cheese, crumbled
- 2 tablespoons black olive paste
- ¼ cup mint, torn

Directions:

2. In a bowl, mix the olives paste with the rest of the ingredients except the cherry tomatoes and whisk well.
3. Stuff the cherry tomatoes with this mix, arrange them all on a platter and serve as a snack.

Nutrition:

Calories: 136,

Fat: 8.6,

Fiber: 4.8,

Carbs: 5.6,

Protein: 5.1

Vinegar Beet Bites

Preparation Time: 10 Minutes

Cooking Time: 30 Minutes

Servings: 4

Ingredients:

- 2 beets, sliced
  Sea salt and black pepper
- 1/3 cup balsamic vinegar
- 1 cup olive oil

Directions:

1. Spread the beet slices on a baking sheet lined with parchment paper, add the rest of the ingredients, toss and bake at 350 degrees F for 30 minutes.
2. Serve the beet bites cold as a snack.

Nutrition:

Calories: 199,

Fat: 5.4,

Fiber: 3.5,

Carbs: 8.5,

Protein: 3.5

Lentils Stuffed Potato Skins

Preparation Time: 10 Minutes
Cooking Time: 30 Minutes
Servings: 8
Ingredients:

- 16 red baby potatoes
- ¾ cup red lentils, cooked and drained
- 2 tablespoons olive oil
- 2 garlic cloves, minced
- 1 tablespoon chives, chopped
- ½ teaspoon hot chili sauce
- Salt and black pepper to the taste

Directions:

1. Put potatoes in a pot, add water to cover them, bring to a boil over medium low heat, cook for 15 minutes, drain, cool them down, cut in halves, remove the pulp, transfer it to a blender and pulse it a bit.
2. Add the rest of the ingredients to the blender, pulse again well and stuff the potato skins with this mix.
3. Arrange the stuffed potatoes on a baking sheet lined with parchment paper, introduce them in the oven at 375 degrees F and bake for 15 minutes.
4. Arrange on a platter and serve as an appetizer.

Nutrition:

Calories: 300,

Fat: 9.3,

Fiber: 14.5,

Carbs: 22.5,

Protein: 8.5

www.ingramcontent.com/pod-product-compliance
Lightning Source LLC
Chambersburg PA
CBHW070735030426
42336CB00013B/1980